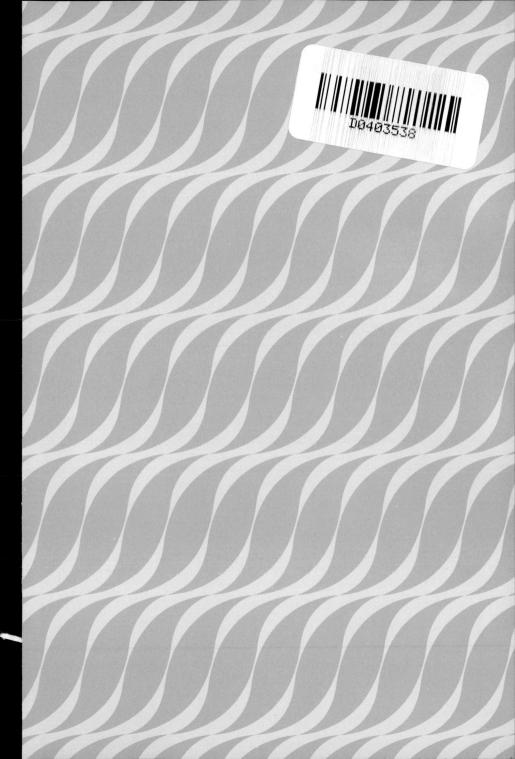

healing with

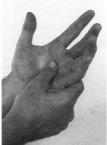

reflexology

a concise guide to

foot and hand massage

for enhanced health

and wellbeing

southwater

Southwater is an imprint of
Anness Publishing Limited
Hermes House
88–89 Blackfriars Road
London SE1 8HA
tel: 020 7401 2077
fax: 020 7633 9499

Distributed in the UK by
The Manning Partnership
251–253 London Road East
Batheaston
Bath BA1 7RL
tel: 01225 852 727
fax: 01225 852 852

Distributed in the USA by
Anness Publishing Inc.
27 West 20th Street
Suite 504, New York, NY 10011
fax: 212 807 6813

Distributed in Australia by
Sandstone Publishing
Unit 1, 360 Norton Street, Leichardt
New South Wales 2040
tel: 02 9560 7888
fax: 02 9560 7488

1 3 5 7 9 10 8 6 4 2

Publisher: Joanna Lorenz
Managing Editor: Helen Sudell
Project Editor: Melanie Halton
Designer: Jane Coney
Photographers: Nick Cole, Michelle Garrett,
Alistair Hughes, Don Last and Liz McAulay
Illustrator: Michael Shoebridge
Production Controller: Joanna King

Publisher's note:

The reader should not regard the recommendations, ideas and techniques expressed and
described in this book as substitutes for the advice of a qualified medical practitioner or
other qualified professional. Any use to which the recommendations, ideas and techniques
are put is at the reader's sole discretion and risk.

contents

INTRODUCTION 4

how does reflexology work? 6

benefits & effects of reflexology 10

getting started 14

massaging the feet 16

reflexology techniques 20

the full reflexology routine 24

SEQUENCES 30

starting the treatments 32

energizing sequences 34

energy boosters 36

improving skin, hair & nails 38

invigorating the immune system 39

enlivening the muscles 40

pain-relieving sequences 42

easing colds, sore throats & sinuses 44

headache relief 46

alleviating menstrual symptoms 47

backache easers 48

repetitive strain relievers 49

digestion improvers 50

relaxation sequences 52

neck & shoulder relaxers 54

stress relievers 56

sleep inducers 58

charts 60

index 64

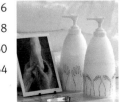

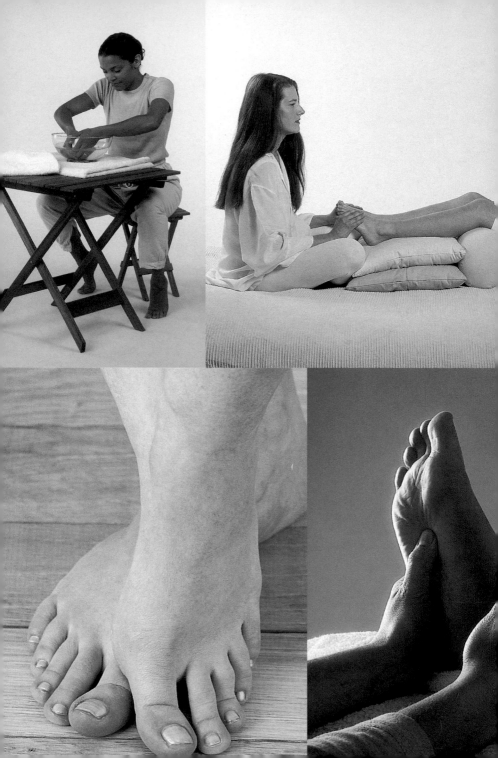

introduction

Our hands have been a means of caring and comforting since we first ceased to need them to walk on and started to use them for focused, specialized activities. Using our hands to release tension in our bodies is something we do instinctively. In reflexology you can use your hands, specifically your fingers, to apply pressure-point therapy to certain points: usually on the feet, often on the hands. The word "reflex" means to reflect. Pressure points on the feet and hands reflect all the parts of your body, both external and internal: organs and glands, as well as limbs, torso and head.

How does reflexology work?

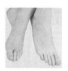 **Reflexology acts on parts of the body by stimulating the corresponding reflexes with compression techniques applied with the fingers. Where the body's functioning is sluggish, we find congestion that has not been cleared away.**

Places on the feet where there are congestion deposits that have not been cleared away by the venous circulation and the lymph will feel tender, sensitive or positively painful; or they may feel hard, tight or lumpy, or like little grains. If these can be worked with massage and compression techniques so that they begin to disperse, the corresponding body part will be stimulated and enabled to heal itself.

HOW THE FEET MIRROR THE BODY
Both feet together hold the reflexes to the whole body. The part that corresponds to the spine therefore runs down the medial line along the instep (the inner edge) of each foot. It will be useful to refer to the charts at the back of the book, as they show the inside body parts in each area of the feet.

▾ WORKING ON THE HEEL AREA FOR THE PELVIS.

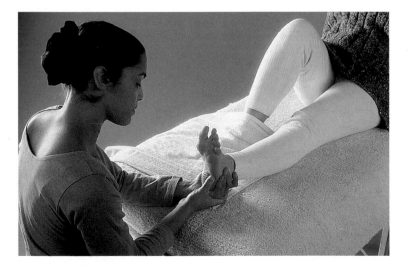

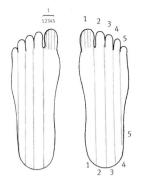

◀ THIS DIAGRAM SHOWS THE FEET ZONES RUNNING ALONG THE FEET. THE BIG TOES REPRESENT THE WHOLE HEAD, AS WELL AS LYING IN ZONE 1. THE RIGHT SIDE OF YOUR BODY LIES ON YOUR RIGHT FOOT, AND THE LEFT SIDE OF YOUR BODY ON THE LEFT FOOT.

HEAD AND NECK

Your head is represented on the toes; the right side of your head lies on the right big toe and the left side on the left big toe. In addition to the whole head being represented on the two big toes, the eight other toes hold the reflexes to specific head parts.

Your neck reflex is found in the "necks" of all the toes: if you find tension in one area of your neck, you will also find tension in the corresponding areas of your toes.

TORSO AND SPINE

It is easy to comprehend how the torso fits on to the body of your feet once you have grasped the concept of your feet representing your whole body. Remember that the spinal line runs down the insteps of your feet.

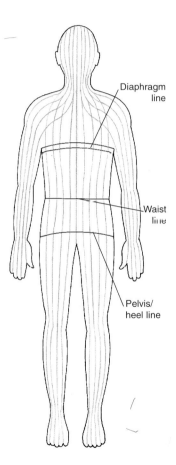

Diaphragm line

Waist line

Pelvis/ heel line

▲ THE ZONES RUN VERTICALLY THROUGH THE BODY, FROM HEAD TO FEET AND HANDS, FIVE ON EACH SIDE. THERE ARE ALSO TRANSVERSE LINES MARKING THE AREAS OF THE BODY.

how does reflexology work? **7**

ABDOMEN

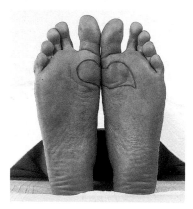

CHEST

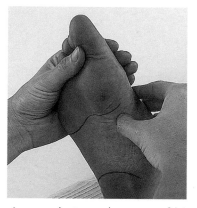

The ball of each foot represents one side of the chest. In the balls of your feet, and on the same area on the top of your feet, lie the reflexes to your lungs, air passages, heart, thymus gland, breast and shoulders. The area is bounded by your diaphragm, as shown right.

In your instep, where your feet are not weight-bearing and so not padded like the ball, are contained all the reflexes to your abdominal organs – those concerned with digestion and the maintenance of life. This area is bounded by the diaphragm line above and by the heel line below.

PELVIS

The whole of your heel all around your foot contains the reflexes to the pelvic area: they lie on the sole and the sides of your heel and across the top of your ankle.

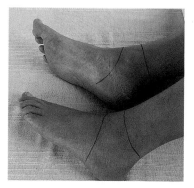

The limbs are represented on the outer edge of your foot but also, and most particularly, on the corresponding upper or lower limb.

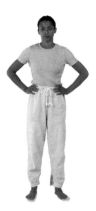

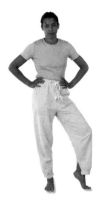

The shoulders and hips reflect each other.

The elbows and knees are related to one another.

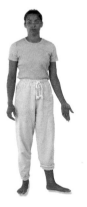

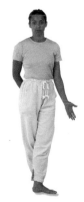

Work the wrist for ankle problems, and vice versa.

Hand and foot are cross reflexes for each other.

Benefits & effects of reflexology

Reflexology works to relax muscle tension. During a treatment all parts of the feet are stimulated to relax muscles and increase the circulation to the body. The effect of this is to achieve a deep state of relaxation.

Working along holistic principles, reflexology takes into account body, mind and spirit as these are all interrelated. Whatever happens to you will affect all levels of your being, whether you notice or not. If you feel under pressure or stressed, the effect on your body will be detrimental as your muscles remain tense and taut, constricting the circulation and nerves, and compromising their functioning. Similarly, if you have a physical mishap your feelings will be affected by the pain you experience, the way the accident

▼ THROUGH WORKING THE HANDS (OR FEET) YOU ARE WORKING THE WHOLE BODY.

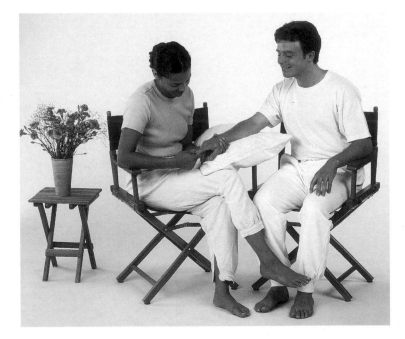

happened, and the effect it has on you afterwards. Although you are working mostly on the feet in reflexology, you are affecting the whole of the body, both inside and out, through the treatment. This is achieved by working the reflexes to the internal organs and glands as well as to the surface of the body. It appears that you can have a more far-reaching effect by working the reflexes than by working directly on the corresponding body part.

Pain in the back, for instance, may be due to a structural problem in which the bones are actually out of place and should be checked by a cranial osteopath, an osteopath or a chiropractor. If the pain results from muscular problems, or if manipulation has already been done but muscular strain remains, the next step is to identify the muscles involved and work to relieve the situation with massage and reflexology.

Reflexology uses both massage and specific stimulation of the reflexes to gain lasting relief from pain. Longer-term benefits result from working the reflexes to the relevant area of the back rather than from working directly on those muscles concerned. This is because through the reflexes you are stimulating the body from within, rather than exercising and soothing the muscles from outside, as with massage. Stimulating the reflex to a troubled area promotes healing.

benefits & effects of reflexology **11**

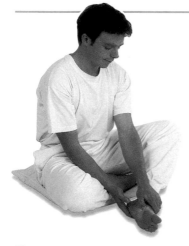

◀ WORKING ON THE SPINAL REFLEX THAT RUNS ALONG THE INSTEP OF EACH FOOT.

THE TREATMENT

Reflexology is not foot massage, but this is incorporated. Sweeping whole hand movements on the foot will relax the patient and prepare the feet for reflex work. During the working of the reflexes, massage soothes and relaxes the area where congestion or discomfort is found. It links the treatment together and relaxes and stimulates the whole body while individual parts are being treated specifically. The use of whole hand massage movements gives a feeling of wellbeing to the entire person.

A reflexology session can be both relaxing and stimulating for the patient. As muscle tensions are relaxed, and the nerve supply freed from constriction, the body slips into a deep state of relaxation. At the same time, the circulation is being stimulated to

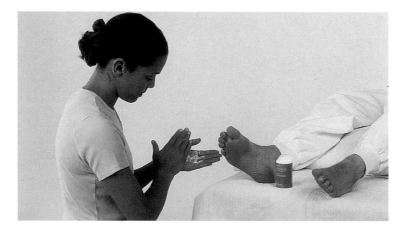

▼ POWDER LIGHTLY DUSTED ON TO YOUR HANDS WILL PREVENT THEM FROM STICKING.

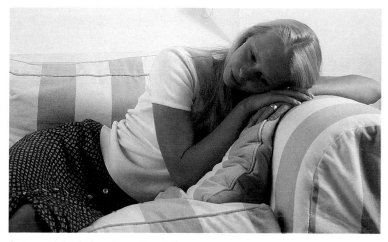

bring nutrients to all parts of the body and to remove waste products and toxins that interfere with the healthy functioning of the parts and the whole. Energy is able to flow more freely around your body, and the functioning of the systems is thus optimized.

TOXINS AND THE HEALING REACTION

Where there are waste products to be cleared from the body, you may experience a healing reaction to treatment, which may take the form of a runny nose, increased perspiration or urination, or increased bowel movements. This reaction represents a loosening of body tensions and is evidence of improved functioning.

▲ YOU MAY FEEL DEEPLY RELAXED AFTER A REFLEXOLOGY TREATMENT.

CAUTION

It is imperative that you only try reflexology on people who are healthy. If you wish to give reflexology to someone without a medical condition but who seems unwell, or who has one of the everyday discomforts described in the sequences in this book, it is important that they should receive professional help before you do anything at all. If you are then able to give some reflexology you must still proceed with caution to safeguard against mishap.

If pregnant, do not work any of the reflexes shown without consulting a reflexologist.

Getting started

Make sure that the room you are going to use for treatment is warm and that you may be quiet in there without interruptions from the telephone, people coming in and going out, or restless pets.

Find a comfortable position for the person whose feet you are going to be treating. They may be propped up along a sofa with cushions to support their back, or sitting in an armchair with an upright chair or stool of a suitable height to support their legs, with a cushion underneath them. Alternatively, you can position your partner on the floor (see below). Make sure that their back, neck and head are fully supported so as not to place the spine under any strain, and that the knees are bent so that the circulation can flow freely.

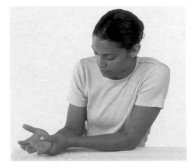

▲ SUPPORT YOUR ARMS WHILE YOU DO REFLEXOLOGY ON YOUR HANDS.

If a partner has sore feet and you are going to work on their hands, it is easier to learn the reflexes if you sit side by side. To work on yourself, find a position that is comfortable.

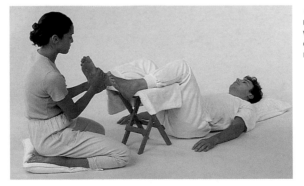

◄ POSITION YOUR PARTNER'S FEET WHERE YOU CAN COMFORTABLY REACH THEM.

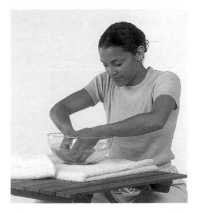

▲ WASH YOUR HANDS IN SOAP AND WATER.

EQUIPMENT

Whichever position you use, you will need to have plenty of pillows to support the back, neck and head. A pillow should be placed under your partner's knees so that they are bent.

Have a blanket or cover ready in case your partner needs extra warmth – their body temperature may drop as they relax.

You will need some towels: one to place under the feet and a couple more for the foot you are not working on to cover it and keep it warm.

Have some powder or arrowroot in case you find that your hands stick to the skin of the feet as you work, if much heat is released. Arrange a pile of cushions, a big cushion or a low stool to sit on as you work. You need to be able to reach and see the feet comfortably without bending over from too high above them. It is very important that you are comfortable: becoming strained or tired will not be good for you, and you may not pay attention properly and could risk doing some damage to your partner.

Before you begin treatment, wash the feet or hands in soap and water. Alternatively, if you have and use essential oils, use a small bowl of water and add a couple of drops of lavender and one of tea tree oil to cleanse them.

▼ ALTERNATIVELY, CLEANSE YOUR HANDS WITH LAVENDER, TEA TREE OIL AND WATER.

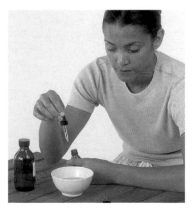

Massaging the feet

It is of great benefit to the patient if the feet are massaged at the beginning of a reflexology treatment to introduce your patient to touch. You should also massage in between reflex work, and to complete the treatment.

To begin

Massage prepares the feet for reflex work: it warms and relaxes the tissues, accustoms the receiver to your touch and soothes and relaxes the whole body. Massage stimulates the receiver's blood supply to and around the feet so that when the reflex points are worked the tissues can respond fully.

During treatment

Use plenty of massage to link the movement from one reflex area to the next, to soothe and relax the foot in between working the reflex points, and use it where any tenderness or discomfort is found.

To complete

When you have covered all the reflex points, end with some whole hand massage on both feet to instil a sense of relaxation.

The massage movements

There is no set sequence for these movements. When you have learnt them, fit them together in a way that feels good to you and adapt them for the individual you are working with as you feel is appropriate. The first few are good as an introduction, and you should always rotate the ankles as this frees up the blood and nerve supply through the ankle to the foot.

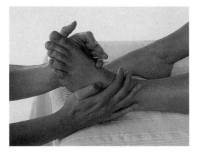

Effleurage or stroking

These gentle movements are just as they sound – sweeping and soothing – and are good to do all over the foot. Add some effleurage movements wherever it feels appropriate throughout the treatment.

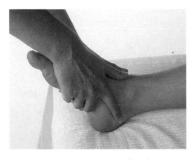

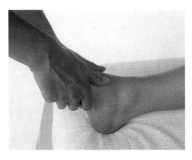

1 Draw your thumbs off sideways, keeping your fingers still.

2 Repeat first movement, working down the foot with each repetition.

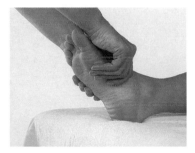

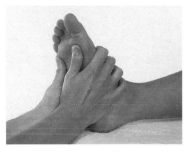

3 To cover the sole of the foot, draw your fingers off sideways, keeping your thumbs still.

4 Finally, massage into the ball of the foot with your thumbs.

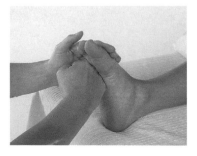

KNEADING

1 Using a similar movement to kneading dough, work into the sole of the foot using the lower section of your fingers, not your knuckles. Use your other hand to support the front of the foot.

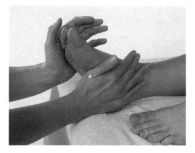

1 These movements are used to stimulate sluggish tissues. Your two hands move in opposite directions. Massage the sides of the foot, running your hands up and down the length of the foot.

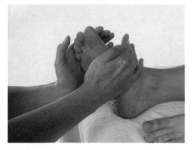

2 Starting at the top of the sole, move your hands alternately up and down. Do not twist the ankle.

ANKLE ROTATION

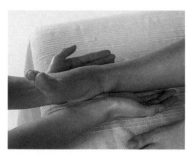

3 With your hands palms up on either side of the foot, move them quickly to and fro to exercise and loosen the ankle.

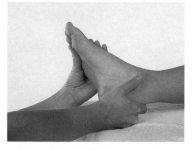

1 Rotate the foot clockwise several times. Never force stiff ankles.

2 Repeat the ankle rotation in an anti-clockwise direction.

Toe rotation

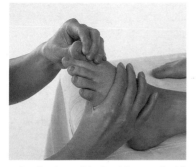

1 Beginning with the big toe, hold the toe securely (not too tightly) and gently rotate it. Repeat this rotating movement with each toe.

Spinal twist

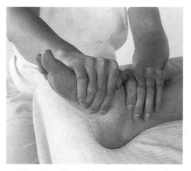

1 The hand on the ankle remains still as the lower hand moves to and fro across the top of the foot, round the instep and back again.

Relaxing your partner

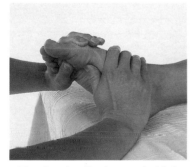

1 To relax the diaphragm, hold the foot with your outside hand, bring the foot down on to the thumb of your other hand and lift it off. Move your thumb to the side; repeat along the ball of the foot.

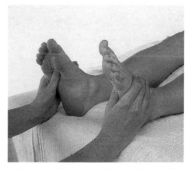

2 To establish good breathing, take both feet and position your thumbs in the centre of the diaphragm line. Press gently with your thumbs as your partner exhales; release as they inhale.

Reflexology techniques

Reflexology works on the whole body, stimulating the reflexes to the internal organs, glands and body parts, as well as massaging the outside of the body. By working on the feet, healing is stimulated through the whole body.

When you have a problem, natural therapies do not address you as a machine – repairing or replacing the part that does not work, regardless of its purpose in the functioning of the whole – but treat you in your entirety to deal with the cause of the problem, rather than merely alleviating the symptoms locally. If you have a raging toothache you may be able to relieve it by taking painkillers, but you will not cause the abscess to go away unless you deal with the poison that gave rise to it in the first place.

If you develop a headache you may or may not know its cause. Where in your body is the trouble seated? Does it come from

▼ USE PILLOWS AS SUPPORT TO MAKE YOUR PARTNER COMFORTABLE.

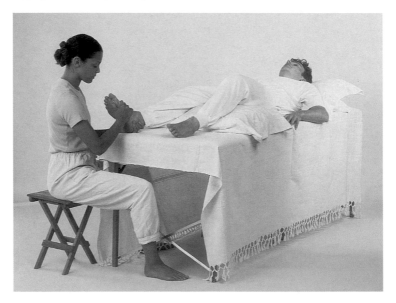

tension in your neck or lower down your spine, from digestive disturbance, or even from held-in tension in your legs? Many headaches have such roots even though we do not notice the beginning of the trouble until a pounding in our head attracts our attention. Recurrent headaches happen because their causes have not been recognized and dealt with. The headache does not really go away, even if it is temporarily relieved by taking painkillers.

If you were to gently massage the reflexes to the head you might be able to give temporary relief from the pain, but you would probably not get rid of the headache. Pressing a reflex point for pain relief is helpful, but short-lived. Stimulating a related reflex, usually more than one, which shows congestion or imbalance, on the other hand, is highly effective in the long term. You will only be able to find these if you work the whole of the feet, rather than spot-working for a specific symptom.

CAUTION

Picking out certain reflexes in isolation is only really effective in the context of working the whole. If you learn and use the routine that follows you will be able to use the sequences in the next section to great effect as part of a reflexology treatment. If you try to bring about a change using only the sequences, you are likely, at best, to be disappointed in the results and, at worst, to aggravate the problem.

▶ THE CAUSE OF AN ACHE MAY NOT LIE WHERE THE PAIN IS FELT.

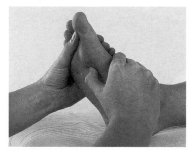

Holding and support

Always use one hand to hold the foot or hand you are working on securely. Position your holding hand near the working hand, not at the other end of the foot, as this can feel insecure.

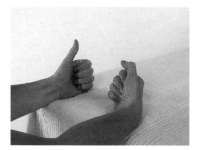

Thumbwalking

1 Hold your two thumbs straight up in front of you and bend one at a time at the first joint. Repeat this movement so that the thumb rests on the skin and travels along its surface.

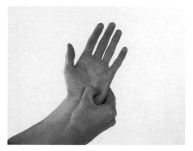

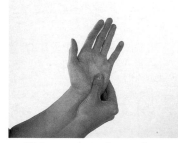

2 The therapeutic movement is on the downward press with your thumb bent. As you do this, put emphasis on pressing down on the skin. Use one hand only: the other holds and supports the foot or hand you are working on.

3 Slide or skate forward as you straighten your thumb. You will still put some pressure on the surface and maintain contact but you are primarily involved in moving forward. This technique is also called caterpillar walking.

FINGERWALKING

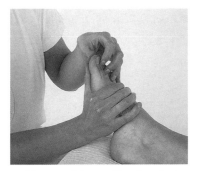

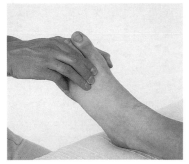

1 Fingerwalking with the index finger. This technique is the same as thumbwalking, but using one or more fingers.

2 Fingerwalking with the three middle fingers together.

ROTATING

PINPOINTING

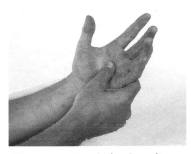

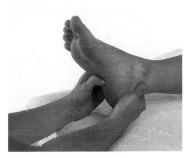

Place your thumb (or finger) on a part of your hand or foot and gently rotate it on the spot. Try exerting a little more pressure. Use this technique when you want to work a specific point.

With your hand in mid-air, move thumb and fingers together and then apart like a pincer. Place your hand on the foot and, with the inner corner of your thumb, press down into the tissues.

The full reflexology routine

The following pages are a step-by-step illustration of the full reflexology routine, which should be performed on your partner before moving to treat specific problem areas. Treat the areas of the body in the same order as shown.

MASSAGE

Begin with some massage and incorporate massage movements into the whole routine, between every area and when you find a tender place. Give a thorough massage at the end to complete.

RIGHT FOLLOWED BY LEFT

The routine is described for one foot. Keep the other warm by covering with a towel. Begin with the right foot and, when you have completed it, duplicate what you have done (reversing hands and movements as appropriate to the shape of the left foot). At the end of the routine you will have followed the diagram on both feet.

◀ ▼ EACH NUMBER (I.E. AREA OF THE BODY) HAS SUBSECTIONS MARKED BY LETTERS AND THE ARROWS INDICATE THE DIRECTIONS OF MOVEMENT.

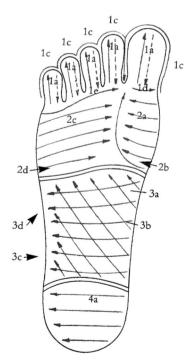

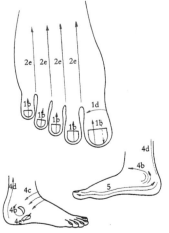

THE SPINE

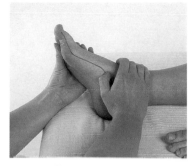

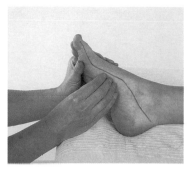

1 You will find the spine running along the instep of the foot. Start or finish the full reflexology routine with these steps. Thumbwalk up the spinal line. Then thumbwalk down it.

2 Use the three middle fingers to fingerwalk across the spine/instep in stages, from big toe to heel.

THE HEAD AND NECK

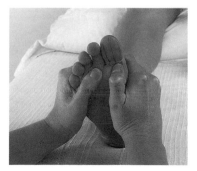

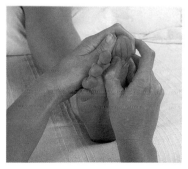

1 The toes refer to the head and neck. Thumbwalk up the back of the big toe, and fingerwalk down the front, in three lines.

2 Thumbwalk up the outside of the big toe. Approach the other side from the back, thumbwalking up the side of the neck. ▶

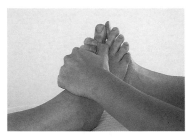

3 Using your other thumb, work up this side to the top.

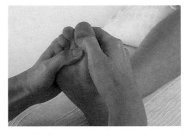

4 Find the centre of the whorls of the big toe print and press gently.

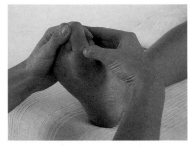

5 Work around the neck of the big toe in a semi-circle.

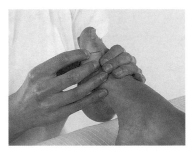

6 Fingerwalk around the front of the big toe with your index finger.

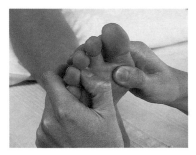

7 Repeat for the smaller toes. Thumbwalk up the back and sides.

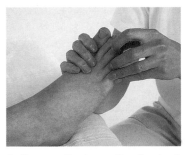

8 Fingerwalk down the front of each toe to its base.

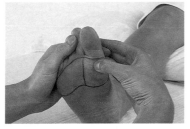

1 Thumbwalk horizontally in from the instep under the big toe.

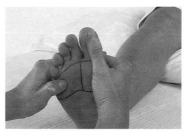

2 Thumbwalk in from the outside of the foot under the little toes.

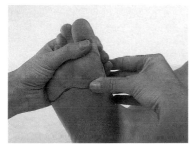

3 Starting just under the big toe, thumbwalk the diaphragm line.

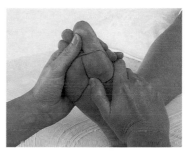

4 Work along the diaphragm line from the inside, up to the toes.

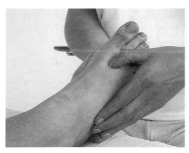

5 Thumbwalk the channel between the bones leading to the toes.

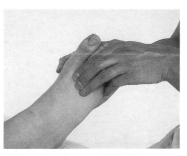

6 Use the three middle fingers to fingerwalk the top of the foot.

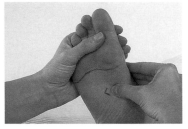

1 Walk horizontal lines from the inner to the outer edge.

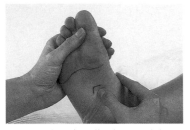

2 Next thumbwalk diagonal lines covering the same area as in step 1.

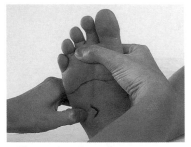

3 Change hands and repeat step 1.

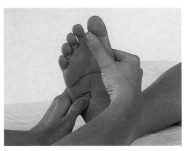

4 Finally, walk diagonal lines from the outside to the inner edge.

THE PELVIS

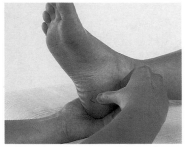

1 Thumbwalk across the heel.

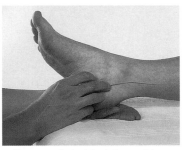

2 Fingerwalk behind the ankle.

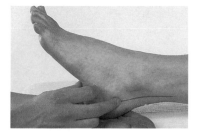

3 Fingerwalk up behind the ankle on the outside.

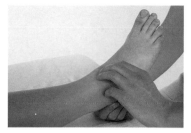

4 Walk across the top of the ankle with three middle fingers.

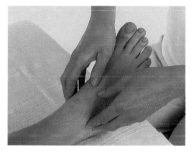

5 Work around the ankle bones with the fingertips.

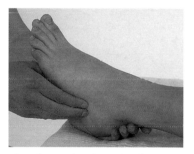

6 Refer to the foot charts at the back of the book to find the hip/knee reflex, and work it by fingerwalking two fingers together.

THE LIMBS

1 Work the outside of the foot, then massage the relevant cross reflex. Now repeat this whold sequence on the left foot having covered the right to keep it warm.

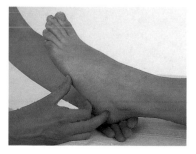

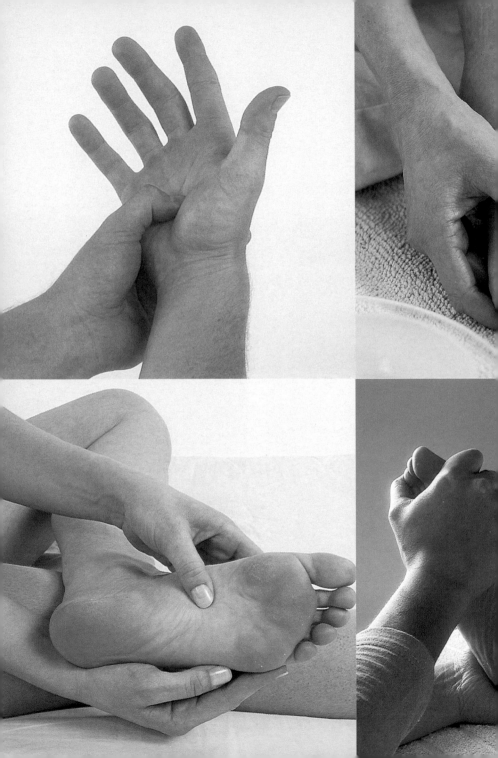

sequences

When you have learnt, and feel comfortable with, the whole routine for giving reflexology, you may begin to pay special attention to treating certain reflexes for specific reasons, as you work. These could include sequences for relaxation, as well as for enlivening muscles, enhancing sleep and energy levels, relieving stress, aches and pains, improving the digestion, strengthening the immune system, and improving skin, hair and nails. When working these sequences, always work the reflex on both feet unless the right or left foot is specified, and be sensitive to the response of your partner.

Starting the treatments

Your way of working the sequences of reflexology must be dictated by the response of your partner, taking into account how they feel, how they are experiencing the massage and what they and you can feel on their feet.

If you are giving reflexology at the end of the day, to relax someone and promote a good night's sleep, when you get to the reflex for the diaphragm you will be aware that it is particularly beneficial to work that part in order to assist relaxation, and so you will work with special awareness there.

In giving special attention to certain reflexes you may feel drawn to do more massage in

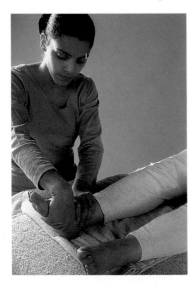

that place, or you may find the reflex is tender and you need to work more gently and perhaps for a little longer to release some of the tension felt there. Or you may stop to rotate on the reflex gently where you would otherwise have covered the area by thumbwalking.

IF YOUR PARTNER FEELS PAIN

Finding congestion or tenderness on the reflexes is never a reason for enthusiastic working at a specific reflex for an extended period, and you must never work if you are causing pain. In this situation massage gently, instead of thumbwalking, and then, if you are able to continue on the tender spot without causing discomfort, do so by working more gently to ensure that you do no harm. The golden rule is that you always take your lead from your partner. Do not go to the other extreme and miss out parts that hurt,

◀ BE SENSITIVE TO YOUR PARTNER'S RESPONSE TO PAINFUL AREAS.

however, as they are just the places that need anything that will assist or stimulate them to heal. Your job is to work out how best you may assist this process and if this means that all you can do without causing pain is to hold the troubled part gently, or just stroke it with a fingertip, you should do so.

As long as you listen carefully to your partner, to what they say and to their body language, and take your approach from what they and their feet are telling you,

▼ POSITION YOURSELF SO THAT YOU HAVE A GOOD VIEW OF THE SOLES OF THE FEET.

CAUTION

Working any of the following sequences in isolation, without working the whole foot routine, will not be effective and may cause damage. These sequences are to add to the basic routine as you work through it.

you will be doing well. Your treatment of the feet will stimulate and balance all of the body systems and you are now ready to incorporate the sequences that follow, if you wish to highlight specific areas.

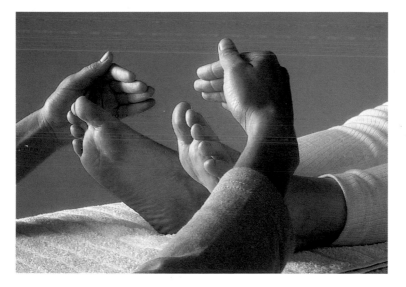

Energizing sequences

To make the most of your potential, your bodily systems need to be functioning well as you start the day and to continue to do so throughout the day. The systems and senses can be stimulated with the following sequences.

INVIGORATING THE BODY

This sequence stimulates all your bodily systems, enabling you to make the most of your potential and start the day in the best way.

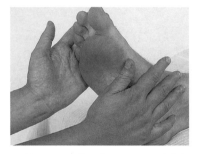

1 Massage the feet to establish good breathing and the instep to stimulate the nervous system.

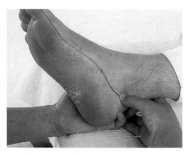

2 Thumbwalk the spine. Rotate the ankles and toes to stimulate circulation and free the nerves.

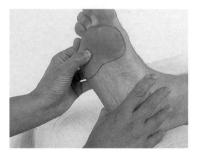

3 Work the diaphragm, and then across the chest to establish deep breathing to strengthen the body.

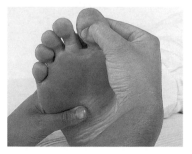

4 Work the pituitary reflex on the big toe in the centre of the toe-print: this is the master gland.

IMPROVING DECISIVENESS

By working the diaphragm, solar plexus and liver you are enhancing good breathing, which improves planning and decision-making.

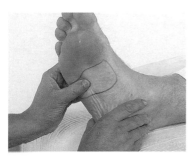

1 Work the liver.

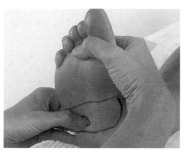

2 Work the gall bladder.

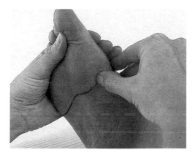

3 Work the diaphragm.

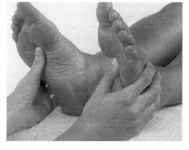

4 Work the solar plexus.

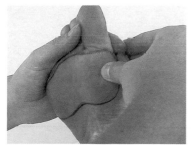

5 Work the lungs.

HELPING HANDS

To aid decisiveness, locate the gall bladder reflex on your right hand and rotate on it with your thumb.

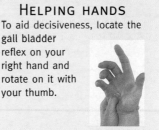

Energy boosters

 If energy is flowing freely around your body you will feel well and find it easier to stay positive. In turn, if you think positively your body will respond and its actions will be enhanced. The power of thought influences physical health and, conversely, your moods are affected by your hormonal balance.

ENHANCING ENERGY LEVELS

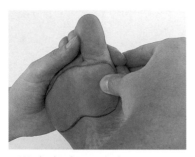

1 Work the lungs to improve your breathing patterns.

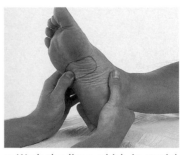

2 Work the liver, which is crucial to your general health.

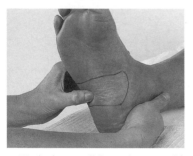

3 Work the small intestines to aid the uptake of nutrients.

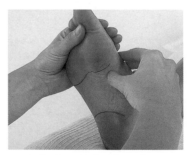

4 Work the whole digestive area. What you eat is turned into your energy during digestion.

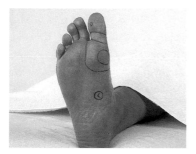

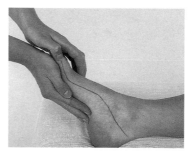

5 Work the glands on the big toe. Rotate the adrenals.

6 Work up and down the spine, your central column of energy flow.

HELPING HANDS

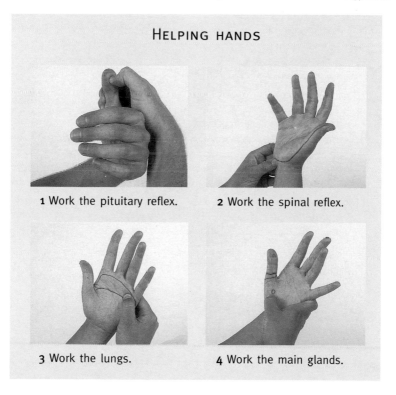

1 Work the pituitary reflex.

2 Work the spinal reflex.

3 Work the lungs.

4 Work the main glands.

Improving skin, hair & nails

To keep your skin, hair and nails in good condition you need hormone balance, good nutrition and effective removal of toxins through the excretory system. Stimulation of the circulation will aid the removal of toxins and the supply of nutrients through the bloodstream.

STIMULATING CIRCULATION

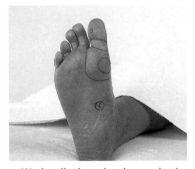 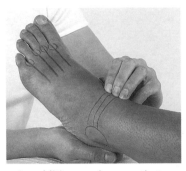

1 Work all the glands on both feet. Your skin, hair and nails are kept in good health by chemicals in your hormones, which are controlled by your glands.

2 In addition, make sure that you give attention to the lymph system on both feet to help remove toxins from the body.

HELPING HANDS

Work all the glands on both of your hands using the chart at the back of the book for easy reference.

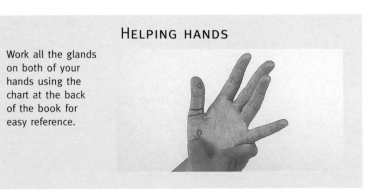

Invigorating the immune system

 Where the immune system is strong, the body will deal naturally with threatening infections so that they cannot become established. Within the context of a full reflexology routine, pay particular attention to the liver, spleen and lymph systems.

IMMUNE BOOSTERS

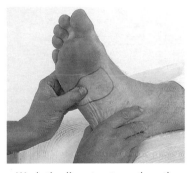

1 Work the liver to strengthen the whole body.

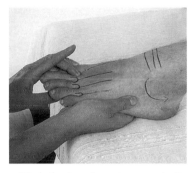

2 Work the lymph systems on both feet to aid the removal of toxins.

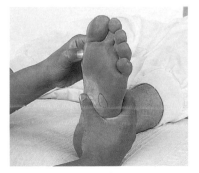

3 Work the spleen (marked on the left foot) and rotate the thymus gland (for both feet) positioned on the ball of the foot.

HELPING HANDS
Work the liver and spleen to strengthen your body, and the thymus gland and lymph system to fight off imminent infection. See the hand chart

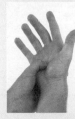 at the back of the book for the specific areas of the hand relating to these parts of the body.

Enlivening the muscles

 A foot treatment stimulates the circulation and all the bodily systems, increasing energy and general wellbeing. If you are doing this reflexology routine for someone else, concentrate on the following areas in your full treatment.

ENERGY ENHANCERS

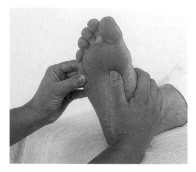

1 Thumbwalk along the line of the shoulders.

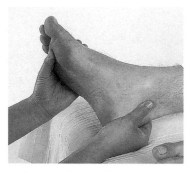

2 Rotate the ankles to loosen tension, increase circulation, and ease pressure on the nerve supply.

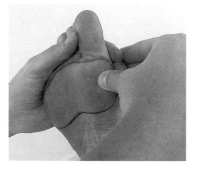

3 Work the whole of the chest and lung area.

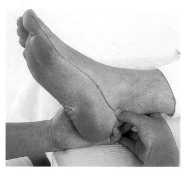

4 Thumbwalk up and down the length of the spine.

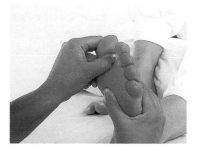

5 Work the neck of all the toes.

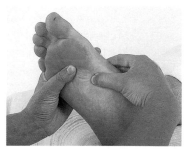

6 Gently rotate the adrenal reflex.

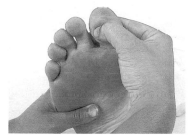

7 Rotate gently on all the reflexes to other important endocrine glands (see step 8) which regulate the chemicals in your body.

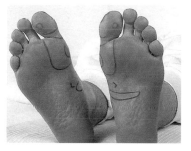

8 Pinpoint the pituitary reflex in the big toe. Thumbwalk the thyroid helper, rotate the adrenals and work the pancreas (left foot).

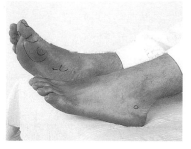

9 Rotate on the ovaries/testes reflex at the side of the heel.

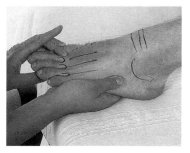

10 Thumbwalk or rotate the reflexes of the lymph system.

Pain-relieving sequences

 If you have not yet read the introduction to the sequences please read it now to make sure that you do no harm. Within a treatment covering the whole of the feet, you may choose to pay special attention to the following areas.

PAIN RELIEVERS

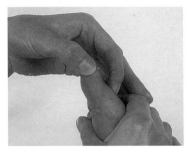

Before concentrating on a specific area of pain, you should work the hypothalamus reflex for the release of endorphins.

PAINFUL MUSCLES OR JOINTS

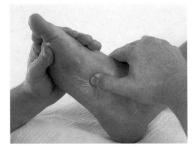

Work the adrenal gland reflexes on both feet. These glands reduce inflammation and aid good muscle tone when working effectively.

BACK PAIN

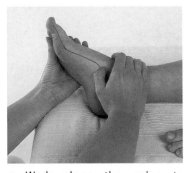

1 Work along the spine to disperse some of the congestion.

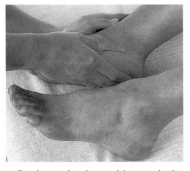

2 For lower back trouble, work the helper area with your thumb.

TOOTHACHE

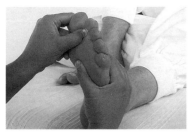

1 Find the toe that has much tenderness and work it carefully.

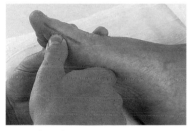

2 Find and carefully work the area of tenderness in the spine.

CRAMP

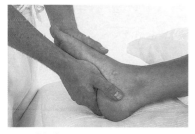

1 Hold the area and massage the appropriate cross reflex.

NERVE PAIN

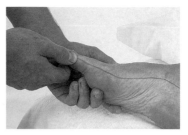

1 Thumbwalk along the spine for the central nervous system.

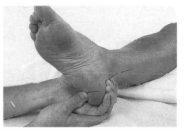

3 For sciatic pain, work the sciatic reflex, as shown.

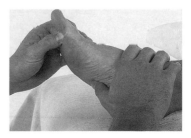

2 Work the parathyroid reflexes round the neck of the big toe.

Easing colds, sore throats & sinuses

Colds, sore throats and sinus problems all affect the respiratory system. To stimulate them to clear themselves of toxins and encourage uptake of nutrients, you need to work all the toes and chest area.

COLDS

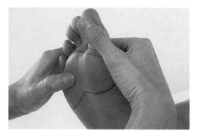

1 Work the entire chest area to encourage clear breathing.

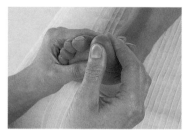

2 Beginning with the big toe, work the tops of all the toes to clear the sinuses. Then pinpoint the pituitary gland in the centre of the prints of both big toes to stimulate the endocrine system.

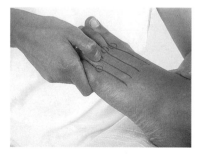

3 Work the upper lymph system to stimulate the immune system.

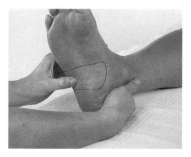

4 Work the small intestines to aid elimination of toxins and uptake of nutrients. Then work the colon to aid elimination. See the chart.

Sore throats

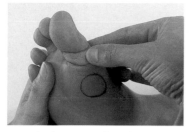

1 Work the upper lymph system, then the throat, and the thymus gland for the immune system.

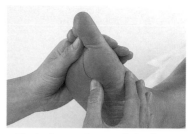

2 Work the trachea and the larynx so as to stimulate them both to clear and heal.

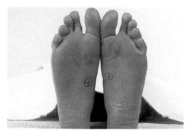

3 Rotate the adrenal reflex in the direction of the arrow.

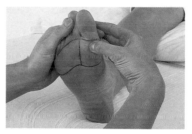

4 Work the thyroid helper in the chest section, then the whole chest area for the respiratory system.

Sinuses

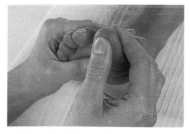

1 Work the sinus reflexes.

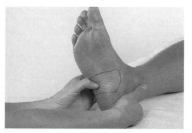

2 Work the ileo-caecal valve.

Headache relief

 Headaches are a common symptom of stress. Often they are caused by tension in the neck and upper back muscles. This can prevent adequate blood supply to the head and thus lead to pain.

TREATING HEADACHES

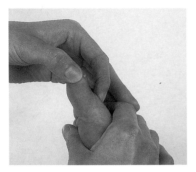

1 Work the hypothalamus reflex first, as this controls the release of endorphins, which help to alleviate pain.

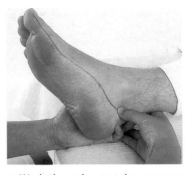

2 Work the spine to take pressure away from the head. This will draw energy down the body and ground it.

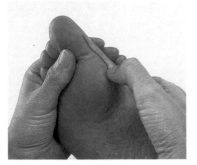

3 Work the cervical spine on the big toe. Work around the neck of all the toes to relieve tension.

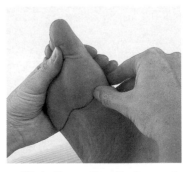

4 Work the entire diaphragm in order to encourage breathing.

Alleviating menstrual symptoms

 Pain during or just before periods is due to contraction in the muscles of the womb which reduces blood flow and causes aching muscles. Work the whole reproductive system on the sides and top of the heel; all parts work together.

MENSTRUAL CRAMPS

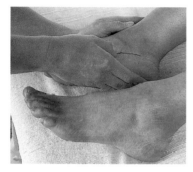

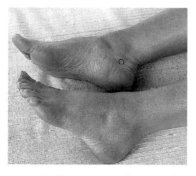

1 Work the lower spine for nerves to the uterus.

2 Work the uterus reflex on the inside of the feet.

PAINFUL BREASTS

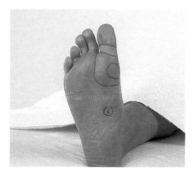

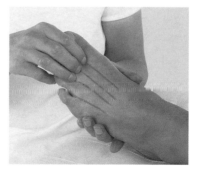

3 Gently work the glands on both of the feet.

Fingerwalk up the chest area on top of the foot holding three fingers together.

Backache easers

Backache is draining, both from the constant aching and because it saps your strength as it constricts your central nervous system (in the spinal cord). Release tension and relax the supporting muscles in the following areas.

EASING TENSION

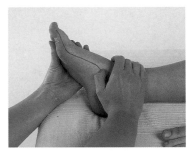

1 Thumbwalk up and down the spine, supporting the outer edge of the foot as you work.

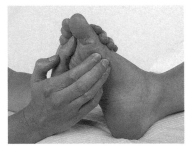

2 Fingerwalk across the spinal reflex with three fingers together, right down the instep in stripes.

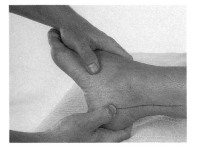

3 Thumbwalk up the helper reflexes for the lower back, behind the ankle bones on either side.

HELPING HANDS
Work the spinal reflex on your own hands.

Repetitive strain relievers

Using a computer for long periods may cause eye strain or your wrists to ache. The best way to relieve repetitive strain is to work the whole feet so that the various systems will be stimulated to function more efficiently.

ALLEVIATING STRAIN

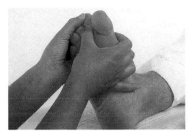

1 Thumbwalk up the second and third toes for the eye reflex.

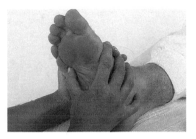

2 Thumbwalk the shoulder reflexes. Fingerwalk the area on the foot top.

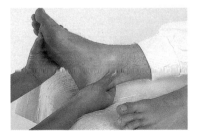

3 Rotate the ankles to ease aching wrists and heal joints.

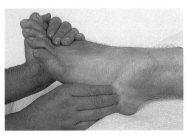

4 Work along the outer foot to relax shoulders, arms and legs.

HELPING HANDS

Use the hand chart to find the relevant reflex on your hands to give temporary, quick relief for your problem. When dealing with repetitive strain, remember that there is no one sequence of movements to help. Work out which part of your body is suffering and locate the relevant reflex.

Digestion improvers

The digestive system is a complex one with many and varied functions. It can easily be affected by tension. In the context of a full reflexology routine, particular attention can be given to the following areas.

INDIGESTION

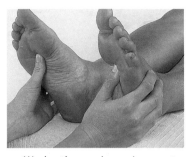

1 Work the solar plexus to relax the nerves to the stomach, then work the stomach, where digestion really begins.

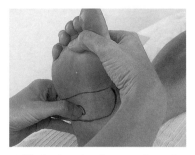

2 Work the duodenum, then the liver and gall bladder: the liver area is shown, with the thumb rotating on the gall bladder reflex.

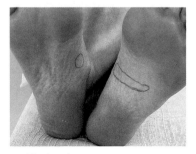

3 Work the pancreas, which regulates blood sugar levels and aids digestion.

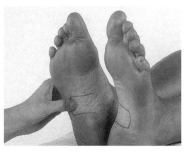

4 Work the small intestines where nutrients are absorbed. If there is bloatedness work the colon. (See the constipation sequence on the opposite page.)

Constipation

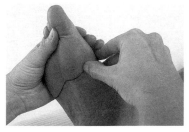

1 Work along the diaphragm to relax the abdomen.

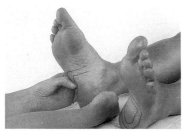

2 Pinpoint the ileo-caecal valve, which links the intestines.

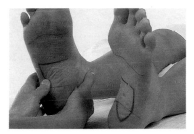

3 Thumbwalk the path of the colon, starting on the right foot.

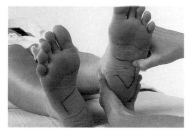

4 Continue on the left foot, using the right hand as above.

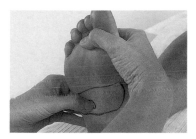

5 Work the liver and rotate the thumb on the gall bladder reflex.

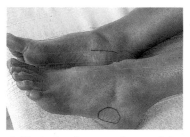

6 Work the lower spine and its helper areas for the nerve supply to the colon.

Relaxation sequences

 Taking time to release built up tension at the end of the day allows your body and mind to unwind and benefit from a good night's rest. Otherwise you may wake stiff, in pain, with a headache or unrefreshed; or you may wake during the night and be unable to get back to sleep.

EASING TENSE MUSCLES

Through massage and stimulating the reflexes you will improve the circulation and this, in turn, will accelerate the body's removal of waste. In this way you are doing what you can to enhance the systems of the body and to enable it to make the most of its healing properties. It is important to use plenty of massage on your partner's feet during the routine. Always include ankle rotation, as this loosens tension there. All the blood supply and nerves to the feet pass through the ankles, and so it is important that these flow freely, unrestricted by excessive tension.

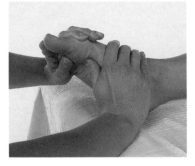

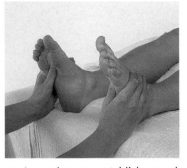

1 To relax the diaphragm, hold the foot with your outside hand, bring it down on the thumb of your other hand and lift it off again. Repeat the movement to work across the foot. Relaxing the diaphragm is important to ease the body and to steady breathing.

2 In order to establish good breathing, take both feet and position your thumbs in the centre of the diaphragm line. Press gently with both of your thumbs as your partner exhales; release as they inhale.

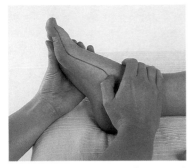

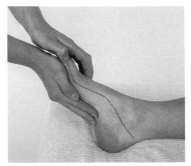

3 Thumbwalk along the spinal reflex from the heel to the big toe. Always remember to support the foot. In this instance, use the other hand to support the outside of the foot.

4 Repeat the movement, going down the spinal reflex. Repeat up and down several times. Slow down to feel for any tight or sensitive parts and rotate gently around those spots.

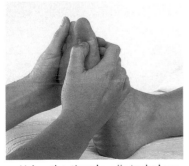

5 Using the thumbwalk technique, work up the back of the toes: do this with care as there is likely to be a lot of tenderness in this area.

HELPING HANDS

You can help to relax tension by massaging the web between your thumb and your index finger on both hands.

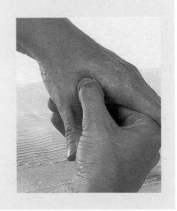

Neck & shoulder relaxers

 We tend to collect a lot of tension in our necks. If you are not aware of neck tension put your hands on either side of your neck and massage gently. If it feels uncomfortable you may benefit from the following sequence, as your partner works your feet.

NECK TENSION

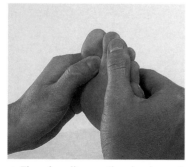

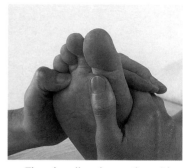

1 Thumbwalk up the back and side of the neck on the big toe. Repeat this on all the toes and thumbwalk around the neck of the big toe, from the back.

2 Thumbwalk along the ridge under the toes. Ensure you are on top of this ridge, as it is easy to move below it, which will not have the same effect.

HELPING HANDS

Thumbwalk along the base of your fingers in order to relax tired, tense neck muscles. This will not only relieve the aching but will also improve tired eyes, and help to reduce any noises in your ears, all of which can be caused by a constriction of nerves in the neck.

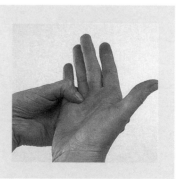

SHOULDER TENSION

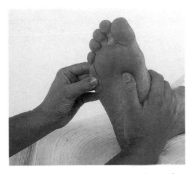

HELPING HANDS
Thumbwalk and massage around the shoulder line on your hands (refer to the hand chart at the back of the book) to relieve the aching caused by shoulder tension. This will also improve your breathing as tight shoulder muscles will pull your chest tight and restrict your breathing.

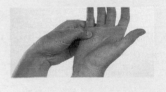

1 To ease tension in the shoulders, thumbwalk along the line of the shoulders in horizontal, overlapping lines. Check the chart.

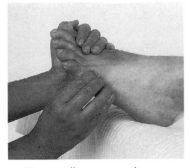

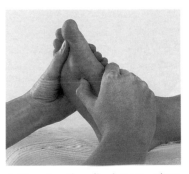

2 Fingerwalk across the same area on the top of the foot with three fingers. Then fingerwalk around the mid-back with three fingers, working in rows from the lower joint of the little toe down to the waistline.

3 To relax the diaphragm, place your thumb on the diaphragm line beneath the big toe. Hold the foot with your outside hand, bring it down on the thumb of your other hand and lift it off again. Repeat to work across the foot.

Stress relievers

When adrenalin levels are high for long periods, the adrenal glands become depleted. Breathing and digestion may be affected. If you feel nervous or queasy, breathe deeply and slowly to increase oxygen supply and calm your nerves.

RELIEVING GENERAL STRESS

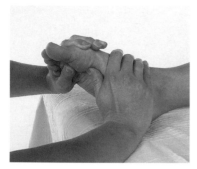

1 Relax the diaphragm, working your thumb across the foot, following the ball of the foot.

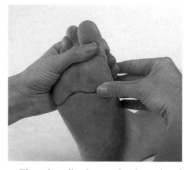

2 Thumbwalk the entire length of the diaphragm line in order to release tension.

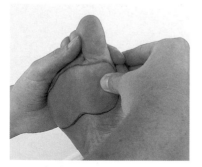

3 Work the lung reflexes on the chest area so that breathing can be increased.

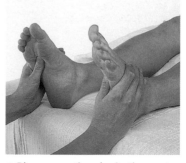

4 Place your thumbs in the centre of the diaphragm line of both feet. Press with your thumbs as your partner breathes out. Repeat.

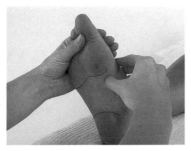

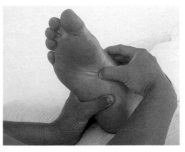

5 Thumbwalk the stomach area and the whole of the instep to help digestion.

6 Use your thumb to rotate gently on the adrenal reflex.

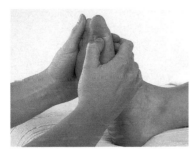

STRESS FROM ANGER

7 Work the neck reflex on the neck of the toes where stress and tension collect.

HELPING HANDS

In order to calm yourself down and settle your nerves, work the solar plexus reflexes and the liver area on your hands for self-help. Refer to the charts at the back of the book as reference.

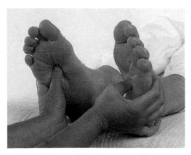

1 Work the solar plexus reflexes on both feet. Then work the liver area.

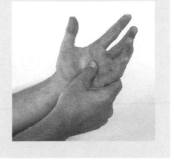

Sleep inducers

 There are many different reasons for insomnia and different manifestations of it. Do you have difficulty in getting to sleep or do you wake during the night? You can help to promote a good night's sleep with this sequence.

SLEEP ENHANCERS

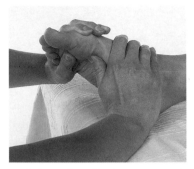

1 Relax the diaphragm: work your thumb across the foot to the outer side, following the diaphragm line.

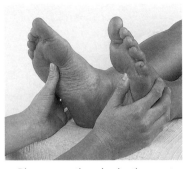

2 Place your thumbs in the centre of the diaphragm line of both feet. As your partner breathes out, press in gently with your thumbs.

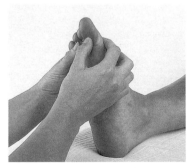

3 Work the neck on all the toes to remove any tension that has built up in the neck muscles.

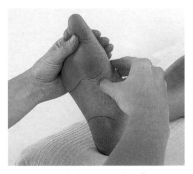

4 Work the abdominal reflexes to relieve tension there.

HELPING HANDS

For self-help gently massage the solar plexus reflex in the palms of your hands.

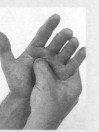

Refer to the hand charts at the back of the book for further information if necessary.

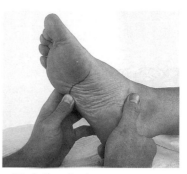

1 Work the diaphragm to promote good breathing.

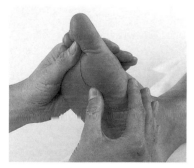

2 Work the air passages in order to stimulate them to clear themselves.

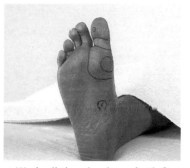

3 Work all the glands on both feet and take particular notice of any that seem especially tender.

HELPING HANDS

Poor diet, smoking and too much alcohol, pollution, toxins and excessive stress are all factors that undermine the body's natural rhythms. Self-help should include a close look at all of the above factors to see how they can be improved.

Foot charts

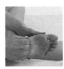

The foot charts are only guidelines for interpretation. When you find a tender part of the foot look for that part on the charts and see which reflex the tenderness lies on. Remember, however, that every pair of feet is different.

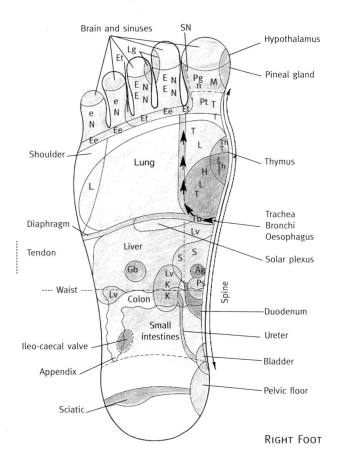

RIGHT FOOT

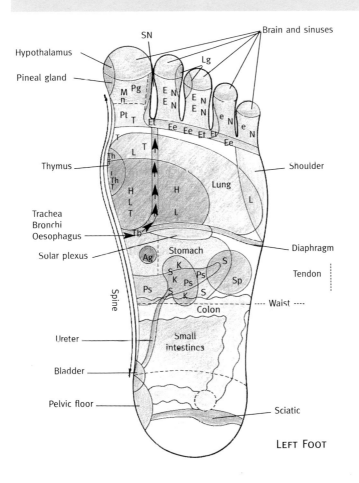

LEFT FOOT

Top & sides of foot

It is not only the soles of the feet that relate to other areas of the body. These diagrams show the areas covered by the tops and sides of the feet. The whole body may be treated on the spinal reflex through the central nervous system.

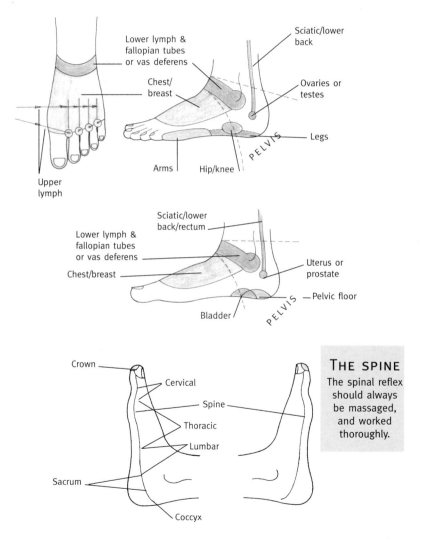

Lower lymph & fallopian tubes or vas deferens

Chest/breast

Sciatic/lower back

Ovaries or testes

Legs

PELVIS

Arms

Hip/knee

Upper lymph

Sciatic/lower back/rectum

Lower lymph & fallopian tubes or vas deferens

Chest/breast

Uterus or prostate

Pelvic floor

Bladder

PELVIS

Crown

Cervical

Spine

Thoracic

Lumbar

Sacrum

Coccyx

THE SPINE

The spinal reflex should always be massaged, and worked thoroughly.

Hand charts

The hands reflect all the body, as do the feet. Once you have adjusted to the basic layout, the location of reflexes is quite straightforward. Use the hand reflexes when you cannot work the feet for any reason.

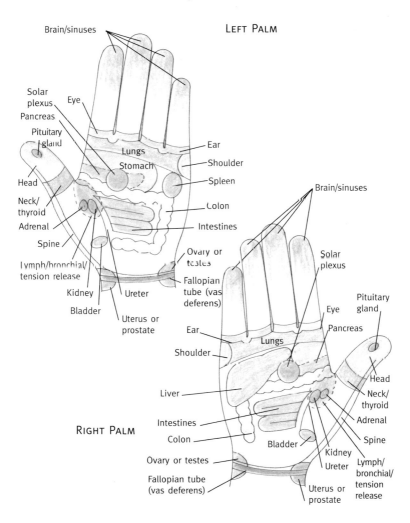

LEFT PALM

Brain/sinuses

Solar plexus
Eye
Pancreas
Pituitary gland
Head
Neck/thyroid
Adrenal
Spine
Lymph/bronchial/tension release
Kidney
Bladder

Lungs
Stomach
Ear
Shoulder
Spleen
Colon
Intestines
Ovary or testes
Fallopian tube (vas deferens)
Ureter
Uterus or prostate

RIGHT PALM

Brain/sinuses

Solar plexus
Pituitary gland
Eye
Pancreas
Head
Neck/thyroid
Adrenal
Spine
Lymph/bronchial/tension release
Ureter
Kidney

Lungs
Ear
Shoulder
Liver
Intestines
Colon
Ovary or testes
Fallopian tube (vas deferens)
Bladder
Uterus or prostate

index

abdomen, 8, 28
anger, 57
ankles, 9

back pain, 11, 42, 48
breathing, 44, 45, 59

chest, 8, 27
colds, 44
constipation, 51
cramp, 43

decisiveness, 35
diaphragm, 52
digestion, 50–51

elbows, 9
energizing sequences, 34–41
energy boosters, 36–7
enlivening muscles, 40–41
equipment, 15

fingerwalking, 23

hair condition, 38
hands, 9, 63
head, 7
headaches, 20–21, 46
healing reactions, 13
hips, 9

immune system, 39
indigestion, 50

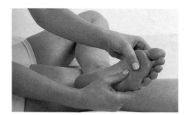

knees, 9

legs, 9

massage, 11–12, 16–19, 24
menstrual problems, 47
muscles, 10–12, 40–41, 42

nail condition, 38
nausea, 46
neck, 7, 54
nerve pain, 43

pain, 21, 33, 42–3, 46
pain-relieving sequences, 42–51
pelvis, 8, 29
pinpointing, 23
preparation, 14–15

relaxation, 10, 12–13, 52–59
repetitive strain, 49
rotating, 22

sequences, the, 32–59
shoulders, 9, 55
sinus problems, 44–45
skin condition, 38
sleep, 52–3, 58
sore throats, 44–5
spine, 7, 25
stress relievers, 56–7
support, 23

techniques, 20–23
thumbwalking, 22
toes, 25–6
toothache, 43
torso, 7
toxins, 12–13

warm-up massage, 16–19
waste products, 13
wrists, 9

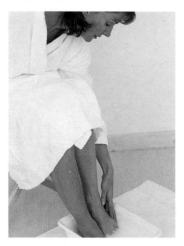

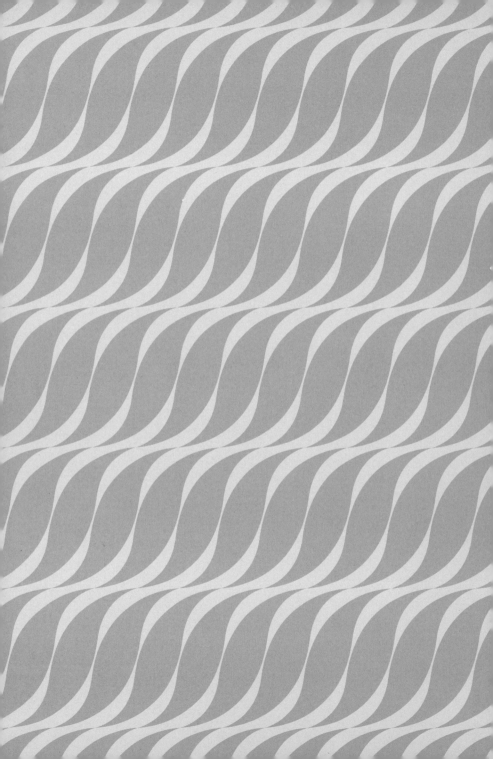